Run

Beginner's Running Program for Distance Made Easy

Table of Contents

Introduction

I want to thank you and congratulate you for downloading the book, *"Run: Beginner's Running Program for Distance Made Easy"*.

This book has actionable information that will help you incorporate running into your life.

Running is undoubtedly one of the oldest workouts known to man and all animals that have limbs. For centuries, man had to run while hunting or to run for his life to escape danger. In recent years, running is part of many sports; Olympics, FIFA World Cup, athletics and many other sporting events.

While running is highly celebrated and even encouraged in everyday life, when many of us think of running, your mind may take you back to your high school gym days. Those days, you were expected to run a certain distance and those who came in last were the butt of several jokes from their classmates. During those times, there was little preparation involved before the actual running took place. Moreover, students ran as fast as they could to avoid coming in last. As a result, they suffered from pains and aches and many of them began associating running with pain or discomfort. Even if you've tried to run in the recent past, you probably either became exhausted too fast, couldn't run for a long distance, felt uncomfortable while running, or were in pain several days after the running session.

This should not be the case. You really don't see the Olympics athletes having expressions of discomfort even after running the marathon. Moreover, you don't need to be running like an Olympics athlete to enjoy the benefits that come with running. You can find joy from running various distances and at various speeds.

This book will show you exactly how to do that. It will show you how to choose the right running gear, the correct running form, warm-up exercises and much more. After reading this book, you will realize that running is not just placing one foot in front of the other.

Thanks again for downloading this book. I hope you enjoy it!

Getting Started: Before You Do Anything Stupid

Get Proper Running Gear

Before you can do anything, it is important that you get the right running gear because this will ultimately determine your comfort level, your running form, the likelihood of injuries and much more.

As far as equipment goes, running does not need specialized equipment. However, you will need running gear especially if you engage in running frequently. So what gear should you get?

1: Sneakers

Running sneakers are the most important part of your running gear. They give you comfort, offer protection and help prevent injury. This is why you may want to get your sneakers from a specialist footwear retailer. Specialized retailers will be able to assess your needs and recommend the best footwear that suits your gait and running style. You can choose from various running shoes. However, before choosing your footwear, it would benefit you greatly to know the wear pattern of your soles. This is what pronation is all about. Pronation refers to the way your foot rolls as the heel strikes the ground. There are three main types of wear patterns that influence the type of shoes you should run in. These are:

- *Neutral pronation* - Neutral pronation is the type of wear shown by biomechanically efficient runners. The wear pattern is centralized in relation to the ball of the foot. The sole also shows some wear at the outer portion of the heel.

Neutral Pronation

If you notice neutral pronation, you will want to purchase neutral footwear. These type of sneakers usually provide shock absorption and arch-side support. You can go for sneakers with extra cushioning for greater shock absorption. Mild pronators can also benefit from using neutral shoes.

- *Overpronation* – This is when the wear is focused on the inside edges of your soles. It shows that your soles roll inwards more than they do with individuals with neutral pronation. Unfortunately, overpronation is often associated with greater risk of injury especially at the knees.

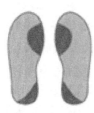

Overpronation

If you exhibit moderate overpronation, you should ask for stability footwear. This type of footwear usually has a 'firm post' that is useful in reinforcing the arch sides of the sneakers. However, if you notice severe overpronation, you would do well to get motion control sneakers. These have stiffer heels and straighter lasts (shape) and are designed to mitigate the effects of overpronation.

- *Supination or under-pronation*

  This is not a common condition with runners. It refers to the way the soles wear along the outer edges. It is characterized by the foot rolling outwards. This means when your foot lands, there will be insufficient impact reduction.

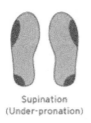

Supination
(Under-pronation)

  If you notice supination or under-pronation, you should get shoes that have extra cushioning and flexibility.

Before purchasing any shoes, you need to make sure you try them out and see how they feel. A good trick is to buy shoes at the end of the day. This is because your feet tend to swell during the day as you carry out various activities. Thus, doing your shopping in the evening will prevent you from buying shoes that don't have extra spacing for your toes.

2: Socks

You will also need a pair of socks. Most runners are comfortable with white sports socks. This is especially so if the socks are designed for running. Such socks wick away moisture and are thick enough to provide extra padding. It would be a good idea to purchase your socks before you purchase your running shoes. This way, you can wear your socks before trying out your shoes to ensure that the fit is right.

3: Shorts and tights

Shorts come in handy when you are running. They are lightweight and they happen to wick away the sweat as you run. You can also wear them when doing other exercises.

Tip: It would be better to get shorts that have a drawstring. This way, you can tighten and loosen the shorts as you wish.

Tip 2: You may also want to add tights to your running gear. They will serve you well during the cold weather.

4: Tops

You will need both short and long-sleeved t-shirts to wear in different weather. You should go for mid to top range tops that have wick away qualities to keep away sweat and ensure you keep cool as you run. Fabrics made from blends of polyester are great at wicking away moisture.

Note: The top you wear should not be too tight or too baggy.

You may want to get long-sleeve t-shirts with cuffed sleeves. This way, the sleeves won't annoy you by riding up your hands. If the weather is very cold, a waterproof top would be best suited for running in.

5: Gloves

It is quite uncomfortable to run when your hands are cold. That's why it may be best to invest in lightweight gloves. You can use woolen gloves since they affordable and will keep you warm in colder weather. However, one disadvantage of woolen gloves is that they don't have waterproof capabilities. Nonetheless, you will be fine if you don't intend to run in wet weather.

6: Watch

Running watches are no longer restricted to stop watches, although you can use that as a beginner. Nowadays, as more and more people turn to running for various purposes, watch designers have become more creative in the watches they create. For example, a GPS watch is used to track things such as time, pace, distance and even calories used among other things. You can get such watches for around $100. If you are serious about distance running, you may want to invest in a GPS watch such as a Garmin Forerunner watch or Fitbit. Alternatively, you can start with a watch that has interval timer features such as the Timex Ironman watch.

7: Sports bra

Many women avoid certain sports simply because they lack adequate support at the bust area. Nobody wants to feel pain whenever their bust moves while running. Thus, it is important for women to invest in a good sports bra. Ensure that the bra fits snugly. However, it should not be uncomfortably tight. You also want to ensure that there are no bulges around the bra sides. Your bust should fit in perfectly.

You may want to try various brands to determine which is best for you.

Note: Always keep your gear clean and ready for use. When the time comes for you to start running you will be ready to go. Before you can become a great distance runner, you need to prepare adequately through stretching. In the next chapter, we will learn why stretching is important before running and what stretching exercises you can to engage in.

Stretching Before Running

Stretching is an issue everyone who engages in some form of exercise has to deal with at some point in his or her life. This is because there are individuals who agree that stretching is important and there are those who frown upon the practice.

Proponents of the practice argue that stretching has a positive effect as far as flexibility is concerned. This is seen clearly in ballet dancers and gymnasts. They engage in a lot of stretching and they are definitely more flexible than most people are. Runners who practice stretching also report increased flexibility. So how does stretching help? Well, for starters, stretching enables your joints to be less resistant to movement. Moreover, it improves muscle coordination and increases your motion range. This comes in handy when you are running especially when you want to pass someone and you have to increase your speed suddenly in order to do so.

However, there are some who oppose stretching. They argue that stretching cold muscles can actually lead to injury. This is because you will be applying force to muscles, which have not been in use. Thus, instead of aiding your workout, stretching can negatively affect your performance as your muscles try to recover from the shock you've given them.

Nevertheless, there is a way you can benefit from stretching. This is by stretching warm muscles. In order to stretch before running, you should:

1: Warm up your muscles

If you've watched the Olympics or other races, you will notice runners running up and down the track and stretching their bodies before their race starts. No, they are not wasting their energy. They are, in fact, warming up their muscles and loosening them up so that they work at their optimal during the actual race. You can warm up your muscles by walking for about five minutes. You can also engage in some light jogging.

2: Stretch your shoulders

When you run, you have to swing your arms. This action puts some stress on your shoulders and you can find your arms getting very tired before you are halfway through your run. This is why you need to loosen up the joints on your shoulder by stretching them. You should begin by rotating your shoulders.

- Place your right fingers on your right shoulder and rotate in for at least 20 seconds.

- Then do the same by placing your left fingers on your left shoulder. Once you are done with each shoulder, rotate both shoulders together.

- Once you've done that, cross your hands above your head such that your left hand is touching your right elbow. Use your left hand to pull your right elbow in the direction of your back. Then change sides.

3: Stretch your back

One of the things you'll notice when you observe people running is that some runners painfully clutch at their backs when they stop running. This is because they feel a lot of tension there. One of the things that causes tension is poor posture. You may unwittingly slouch when sitting or standing. Many runners tend to lean forwards especially when they are tired. This just adds to the tension. You need to make it a point to stretch your back. This will relieve some of the tension and prepare you for a good run. Here's what you should do:

- Stand up straight.

- Push your pelvis upwards while slightly bending your knees.

- Stretch out both of your arms in front of your chest and interlock your fingers with your palms facing outwards.

- Bend your upper back so that it looks rounded and bend your head towards your chest. This position should make you feel a stretch in your back. Hold for a moment and then release.

4: Stretch your chest

Another area you need to stretch is your chest. Depending on your level of fitness, you will experience some discomfort in your chest area as you run. This should ease as you become a regular runner. In order to stretch your chest, you should:

- Stand up straight.

- Place your hands above your butt (on the small of your back). Your elbows should be bent.

- Gently push your elbows together at your back. You will feel your chest stretch. Hold the position for a moment before releasing.

Stretching gets you ready to run. However, you need to improve your running form in order to achieve greater success as far as distance running is concerned.

Improve Your Running Form

Some people make the mistake of thinking that running requires no skill. If this were true, there would be more people running and winning races and fewer people injured because they overused their muscles. A good running form will not only improve your speed and allow you to cover greater distances, but it will also lower your risk of injury. In order to improve your running form you should:

1: Increase your cadence

Many beginner runners make the mistake of thinking that longer strides will help them achieve their goals faster. This is not true. You would do better to keep your cadence to 170-180 steps per minute. Cadence refers to the number of times your feet strike the ground during a particular period of time. It is usually calculated as strikes (steps) per minute. Individuals who record a cadence of 160 steps per minute are most likely over-striding. Track your steps if you don't have a watch to do that for you. This way, you will see whether or not you need to reduce your increase your steps.

Think of it this way. You can only move forward once your foot touches the ground to make way for the other foot to move forward. Thus, the faster your foot touches the ground, the faster you will be able to move. Therefore, it makes sense for you to increase your cadence.

2: Watch where you land

This goes hand in hand with cadence. If you take longer strides, you will be over-striding or overreaching as far as your landing foot is concerned. You need to land with your foot just underneath your body. You should not land as if you are trying to reach a spot in front of you. If you do overreach, you will only be straining your muscles and increasing your risk of injury. Another advantage to landing your foot underneath your body is that you will greatly reduce heel-striking. This means you will be able to increase your speed, as you will be landing on your mid-foot most of the times.

3: Run tall

The only time you should bend from your waist when running is when you are at the finish line and you want to get an advantage over other runners who are at the line with you. This however, is not a book on racing. Otherwise, keep your back straight. Only bend slightly forward from your ankles as you run. Do not slouch even when you are tired.

3: Land on your mid-foot

You need to avoid landing on your heel. Aim at landing on your mid-foot. If you make it a point to land your foot underneath your body, you will begin to land on your mid-foot more and more. But don't be alarmed if you land slightly on your heel. Just shoot for this goal and you will become better at it as you become more experienced.

4: Take note of your arms

As a runner, one thing you need to avoid is swinging your arms across your chest. Instead, keep your arms at about 90degrees as you run. Don't let them fall at your sides and don't hold your back as you run.

Improving your form may take some time especially if you are used to running without much thought to form. You may even find that your running time increases as you try to switch on to the proper running form. Don't become discouraged. Keep at it and you will reap great benefits. Also, ensure that you engage in some stretching exercises once you are done with your running.

Now You Can Run

Stage 1: Walk/Run Technique

The good thing about running is that you are not restricted when it comes to training times or gym times. You get to choose the most convenient time for you to run. However, it is very important that you don't overexert yourself. Distance running requires a certain amount of patience whether you are new to running or whether you've only been running short distances. One very effective method that will enable you to become a successful distance runner is the walk-run technique.

As the name suggests, the walk-run technique involves both walking and running. Beginner runners use this to get into the habit of fulltime running. It is also used by experienced runners who want to increase the distance they run even as they reduce their risk to injury. Let's face it. If you are not used to running long distances, you will be in a lot of pain if you try to cover such distances at one go. The walk-run technique enables you to ease into your running habit. In the foreseeable future, you will be able to increase your mileage and the speed with which you run.

In order to do the walk-run technique, you should:

1: Follow a walk-run pattern

The walk-run technique is designed to enable you to ease into fulltime running. That is, running without stopping to take a walk. As a beginner, you need to start with a walk-run ratio of 7:1. This means taking a walk for 7 minutes before switching to run for 1 minute. You should always start with the walking portion as this will warm up your muscles. You can even do your stretching after you walk for the first time before you start running. An interval watch can help you keep track of when to change up from walking to running.

The walking portion is not an excuse to take a leisurely stroll. Make sure that you pump your arms as you walk and that you keep a quick pace. This will keep your heart pumping and it will be easier on you when you switch to running. Continue switching according to the ratio until you cover the desired distance.

2: Make adjustments to your pattern

You need to continue using the walk-run technique while reducing your walking time even as you increase your running time. For example, if the walk-run ratio is 7:1 in week 1, by week 8 the ratio should be 1:7. Eventually, you should be able to run from start to finish. This means, reducing the minutes you walk and increasing the minutes you run each week until you arrive at your goal. Listen to your body as you make the needed adjustments. If you feel you are moving too fast, slow down instead of pushing yourself too hard.

The walk-run technique is also useful when you want to increase your distance further. Thus, always keep it in mind when you want to make some changes. Remember to drink water before you start and in the middle of your walk-run exercise.

Stage 2: Endurance, Strength, And Stability

Increasing the distance you run is not easy, especially for beginners. It takes a period of adjustment and it has to be done intelligently. If you try to cover too much too soon, you will suffer from burnout, as your muscles will not have the needed time to recover. Here are some steps to help you build up your endurance:

1: Take a step farther

If you are serious about distance running, you will strive to increase your distance each week. However, that is easier said than done. But one way to do it is by taking 'one more step'. This may mean running one street farther or one more corner. The basic idea is to keep on increasing the distance you run even if by a little. However, don't do too much too soon. As a rule, you should only increase your distance by 10% each week. It will add up.

2: Slow down

Sometimes you need to slow down in order to run further. Many runners have found success by just slowing down 30 seconds each mile. Do the conversation test where you maintain a conversational pace when you run. If you find yourself unable to carry out a conversation, you are running too fast. Slow down, increase your distance and eventually you will be able to increase your speed as your body adjusts.

3: Rest

Do not ignore rest days. Your body needs to rest, recover, and rejuvenate in order to be healthy enough to run some more. In fact, you should make it a point to have one full day of rest where you don't do any running or any exercises. Distance running can be done once a week. You can engage in shorter runs twice a week to build your endurance. This will also prevent you from overexerting yourself.

4: Improve your conditioning

Don't just concentrate on running. You need to make it a goal to improve your overall condition. The better shape your body is in, the easier it will become for you to run long distances. Thus, look into including cross training and core workouts into your weekly routine. If you are running 3 times a week, you can work out the other days and put aside one day for rest.

Endurance is about training your body to run longer distances. It does not occur overnight but it can be done through patiently increasing the distance you run each week. Once you have achieved your goal, you can go ahead and work on your speed.

Stage 3: Speed Work

Speed work means exactly that – working on your speed. This is done through interval training whereby you determine a certain distance you want to run. You break the distance into intervals and you run a certain distance at a higher speed than you would normally run and then 'rest' by jogging for a certain period of time before running at the higher speed again. You can do speed work on various surfaces. These are:

- Track

If you are running on a track, one example is to run two laps. When on the straights, run at a higher speed. When you reach the curves, stop running and start walking briskly. Repeat for the two laps.

- Trail

When you are on a trail, you will need to use a watch to see when you need to increase your speed. You will need to do at least 3-4 high speed runs for 20 seconds each. Jog during 'rest' periods.

- Hills

Hills are great for increasing your speed. You start with an easy run and make sure you include 3 20-second runs at a higher pace. Continue the easy run at rest intervals.   Hills are one of the best ways to build conditioning, but you may want to wait until you have some decent experience under your belt.

As a beginner, you can time the amount it takes for you to recover from a higher speed running. This is the time you take to catch your breath normally. Then use that as your 'rest' interval. Don't rest too long and don't stop activity during the rest interval. Your body needs to be able to get back to running as soon as possible and this means keeping your muscles warm.

After Every Run: Stretching After Running

As a runner, you need to develop a habit of stretching your muscles after every race or workout. As you stretch your body, you should focus on the muscles that runners use the most. Thus, your stretching exercise should include:

1: Hamstrings stretch

Tight hamstrings often lead to lower back problems. You definitely don't want to keep dealing with this as a runner. This is why you need to do a hamstrings stretch. You should:

- Lie down on your back.

- Bend your left leg and bring it towards your chest.

- Gently straighten your left leg at a 90degree angle while grabbing it with both your hands at the knee area.

- Pull your leg towards you but keep your hips on the ground. Hold the position for at least 10 seconds before releasing. Repeat on the other leg. However, if you find it too hard to stretch with your leg straight, you can slightly bend the knee of the leg you stretch.

2: Quadriceps stretch

Your hamstrings contract whenever you stretch your quads. This helps them to get stronger. In turn, you find that your speed increases as these are the muscles responsible for lifting your knees. In order to do a quadriceps stretch, you should:

- Stand up straight with your legs hip-width apart. You can place your hand on a chair for support but ensure that you keep your back straight.

- Lift your left leg towards your butt. Extend your left hand backwards to pull your left leg close to your backside. Keep the other leg straight. Hold the position for at least 10 seconds before changing sides.

3: Calf stretch

Calf muscles are important when you want to lengthen your stride and increase your speed. In order to do a calf stretch, you should:

- Find a wall or a tree.

- Stand at least two feet from the wall and put your palms against it. Your elbows should be bent.

- Slide your left leg behind as you straighten your arms. Your right leg should bend at the knee as you do this. You will feel your straight leg stretching at the calf. The further back you push your leg, the more you will feel the stretch. Hold the position for at least 10 seconds before switching sides.

Once you start stretching after your runs, you will notice a difference as far as your flexibility is concerned. Thus, make it a habit to stretch after every run even when you are tempted not to do so.

In the next chapter, we will discuss the role of nutrition in running.

Diet And Nutrition

The food you eat not only keeps you in good health but it also promotes peak performance. Nutrition affects how you feel, your energy levels, and how you think. All these things will determine whether or not you have a successful run. Therefore, you should make it a point to always eat a balanced diet. This includes eating:

Carbohydrates

Carbohydrates are your main source of fuel and they should make up at least 60-65% of your calorie intake. You can eat foods such as brown rice, potatoes, whole grain bread and pasta, fruits and starchy vegetables. Make sure to eat slow release carbs (e.g. whole grain, soup, starchy veggies etc.) when you are not running such as the night before and small portions of fast release carbs (e.g. bananas, oranges, etc.) while you are just about to start running.

Protein

Do not neglect protein. Protein serves the important function of helping your body repair damaged tissues. Given the amount of damage your tissues can undergo during your training, you need to make it a point to include at least 15-20% protein in your daily diet. This means including things such as fish, poultry, dairy products, meats, legumes and whole grains. The timing of your protein intake is also very important. It is best that you take more protein after workout.

Fat, vitamins and minerals

Fat is not your enemy. Your diet should be made of 20-25% fat. Eat foods such as nuts, oils and fish. Fish is well known for providing omega-3 fatty acids that are useful for your health. Apart from fats, you should also make sure you get your fair amount of vitamins and minerals. Vitamins are great antioxidants and thus can help you get rid of toxins as you engage in exercise and running. Minerals such as calcium, iron and sodium are great for runners. Calcium is good for your bones and iron helps deliver oxygen to your body's cells. You may need to increase your sodium intake as this vital mineral is often lost when you sweat. Sports drinks may come in handy in replacing sodium and other electrolytes. Alternatively, you can take salt when you run to help minimize your water loss due to perspiration- salt is high in sodium, which helps the body to retain water. And as always, remember to keep yourself hydrated.

You can learn more about the specific foods to eat with a simple google search.

Before going for runs, you should avoid heavy meals. Instead, take a healthy snack rich in carbs at least an hour before your run. There is no need for you to turn to sugary foods for energy.

Note: Always keep in mind that running does not give you the green light to overindulge. If you take in much more calories than you need, you will begin to store fat (from the surplus calories) and this will eventually interfere with your running. Always maintain a healthy diet and ensure that you work on your mental health.

Mental Marathon

If you've watched a distance race or marathon, you will notice that there are many times young inexperienced runners have been completely outwitted by older experienced runners. As such, don't be surprised when you see older men and women pass you by as you begin your distance running training. This is because distance running is not just about the physical running aspect. It also involves your mental stamina. In order to be successful at distance running, you will also have to win the mental marathon. There are various factors that will influence your running. These are:

1: Internal association

Internal association refers to the way you focus on how your body feels during your training. Many runners make the mistake of focusing on pace instead of listening to how their body feels. The truth is there are many things that can affect your running on any particular day. This includes training fatigue, weather changes, stress, dehydration, or a lack of sleep. You need to be aware of your body. This will enable you to take preventive measures to avoid injuries and slow down your pace as needed; many runners have indeed increased their distance by slowing down. And as their bodies adjusted to running long distances, their speed increased.

2: Internal disassociation

This refers to the distractions that crop up internally as you engage in running. You may find yourself singing along to a song in your head or trying to solve a puzzle or thinking about things you need to do later on in the day. Internal disassociation can help you cover longer distances. However, it is a distraction. And like other distractions, it can blind you to how your body is feeling and what is going on in the environment around you.

3: External association

When you enter a race for example, there are some things you need to be aware of. These include things such as calculating your split times to know how you are doing, being aware of being passed by others, focusing on passing those in front of you and being on the lookout for fluid stations that will help you hydrate. This is external association. It focuses on the external things that are important to the race. As a distance runner, you need to keep such things in mind.

4: External dissociation

When you are racing again for example, there are other things you will notice or hear that are unimportant to the run. These are things such as the scenery, spectators or even the eccentricities of other runners. If you allow yourself to be distracted by beautiful scenery, you will lose ground. As a runner, you must learn how to tune out spectators. Don't start waving at everyone and looking for familiar faces among the spectators. You should also refrain from staring at outrageously costumed runners, as this will slow you down. You need to disassociate from things that are not important to the race. Unless of course, your intention is just to run for fun.

At the end of the day, you need to know what to give attention to as a runner and what to ignore in order to improve how you run.

Conclusion

Distance running can be the most satisfying venture you undertake. However, it requires some planning. You need to ease your way into it, rather than trying to run too far, too fast. Give your body the time to adjust by using the walk-run technique. This way, you will definitely train your body to run fulltime. Also, make sure you wear proper clothing, watch what you eat, hydrate and prepare yourself mentally before running. This will help you to be in top form during your run. Remember also to pay attention to your running form and your cadence and to stretch after your run. If you do all these things, you will find success as a distance runner. This will be a great beginning to your running habit and will hopefully lead to a passion.